Controlled

Drug

Record

LTC/Rehab/AL/CBRF

ISBN: 9781086673234

Controlled Substance Log

Controlled Substance Log

(Page number correlates with log number)

Page #	Resident	Medication	Dose	RX#	Date Received	Nurse	Date Complete
1							
2							
3							
4							
5							
6							
7							
8							
9							
10							
11							
12							
13							
14							
15							
16							
17							
18							
19							
20							
21							
22							
23							
24							
25							
26							
27							
28							
29							
30							
31							
32							
33							
34							
35							
36							
37							
38							
39							
40							
41							
42							

43						
44						
45						
46						
47						
48						
49						
50						
51						
52						
53						
54						
55						
56						
57						
58						
59						
60						
61						
62						
63						
64						
65						
66						
67						
68						
69						
70						
71						
72						
73						
74						
75						

Resident
Record

Resident Controlled Substance Record

<table>
<tr><td colspan="3">Resident</td><td>Date Received</td><td colspan="2">MD</td></tr>
<tr><td colspan="2">Medication</td><td>Dose</td><td>RX#</td><td colspan="2">Nurse receiving</td></tr>
<tr><td colspan="2">Directions for medication (May place pharmacy Label)</td><td></td><td>Amount received</td><td colspan="2">2nd Nurse signature</td></tr>
</table>

#	Date	Time	Amount Given	Nurse Signature	Amount Remaining
1					
2					
3					
4					
5					
6					
7					
8					
9					
10					
11					
12					
13					
14					
15					
16					
17					
18					
19					
20					
21					
22					
23					
24					
25					
26					
27					
28					
29					
30					

Medication Disposition Record

Date: _____ Quantity Destroyed: _____ Quantity sent with resident: _____

Nurse 1: _____

Nurse 2: _____

Comments: _____

Resident Controlled Substance Record

Resident				Date Received	MD
Medication			Dose	RX#	Nurse receiving
Directions for medication (May place pharmacy Label)				Amount received	2nd Nurse signature

#	Date	Time	Amount Given	Nurse Signature	Amount Remaining
1					
2					
3					
4					
5					
6					
7					
8					
9					
10					
11					
12					
13					
14					
15					
16					
17					
18					
19					
20					
21					
22					
23					
24					
25					
26					
27					
28					
29					
30					

Medication Disposition Record

Date: _____ Quantity Destroyed: _____ Quantity sent with resident: _____

Nurse 1: _____

Nurse 2: _____

Comments: _____

Resident Controlled Substance Record

Resident				Date Received	MD
Medication			Dose	RX#	Nurse receiving
Directions for medication (May place pharmacy Label)				Amount received	2nd Nurse signature

#	Date	Time	Amount Given	Nurse Signature	Amount Remaining
1					
2					
3					
4					
5					
6					
7					
8					
9					
10					
11					
12					
13					
14					
15					
16					
17					
18					
19					
20					
21					
22					
23					
24					
25					
26					
27					
28					
29					
30					

Medication Disposition Record

Date: _____ Quantity Destroyed: _____ Quantity sent with resident: _____

Nurse 1: _____

Nurse 2: _____

Comments: _____

Resident Controlled Substance Record

Resident			Date Received	MD	
Medication		Dose	RX#	Nurse receiving	
Directions for medication (May place pharmacy Label)			Amount received	2nd Nurse signature	

#	Date	Time	Amount Given	Nurse Signature	Amount Remaining
1					
2					
3					
4					
5					
6					
7					
8					
9					
10					
11					
12					
13					
14					
15					
16					
17					
18					
19					
20					
21					
22					
23					
24					
25					
26					
27					
28					
29					
30					

Medication Disposition Record

Date: _____ Quantity Destroyed: _____ Quantity sent with resident: _____

Nurse 1: _____

Nurse 2: _____

Comments: _____

Resident Controlled Substance Record

Resident				Date Received		MD	
Medication			Dose	RX#		Nurse receiving	
Directions for medication (May place pharmacy Label)				Amount received		2nd Nurse signature	

#	Date	Time	Amount Given	Nurse Signature	Amount Remaining
1					
2					
3					
4					
5					
6					
7					
8					
9					
10					
11					
12					
13					
14					
15					
16					
17					
18					
19					
20					
21					
22					
23					
24					
25					
26					
27					
28					
29					
30					

Medication Disposition Record

Date: _____ Quantity Destroyed: _____ Quantity sent with resident: _____

Nurse 1: _____

Nurse 2: _____

Comments: _____

Resident Controlled Substance Record

Resident			Date Received	MD	
Medication		Dose	RX#	Nurse receiving	
Directions for medication (May place pharmacy Label)			Amount received	2nd Nurse signature	

#	Date	Time	Amount Given	Nurse Signature	Amount Remaining
1					
2					
3					
4					
5					
6					
7					
8					
9					
10					
11					
12					
13					
14					
15					
16					
17					
18					
19					
20					
21					
22					
23					
24					
25					
26					
27					
28					
29					
30					

Medication Disposition Record

Date: _____ Quantity Destroyed: _____ Quantity sent with resident: _____

Nurse 1: _____

Nurse 2: _____

Comments: _____

Resident Controlled Substance Record

Resident			Date Received	MD	
Medication		Dose	RX#	Nurse receiving	
Directions for medication (May place pharmacy Label)			Amount received	2nd Nurse signature	

#	Date	Time	Amount Given	Nurse Signature	Amount Remaining
1					
2					
3					
4					
5					
6					
7					
8					
9					
10					
11					
12					
13					
14					
15					
16					
17					
18					
19					
20					
21					
22					
23					
24					
25					
26					
27					
28					
29					
30					

Medication Disposition Record

Date: _____ Quantity Destroyed: _____ Quantity sent with resident: _____

Nurse 1: _____

Nurse 2: _____

Comments: _____

Resident Controlled Substance Record

Resident			Date Received	MD	
Medication		Dose	RX#	Nurse receiving	
Directions for medication (May place pharmacy Label)			Amount received	2nd Nurse signature	

#	Date	Time	Amount Given	Nurse Signature	Amount Remaining
1					
2					
3					
4					
5					
6					
7					
8					
9					
10					
11					
12					
13					
14					
15					
16					
17					
18					
19					
20					
21					
22					
23					
24					
25					
26					
27					
28					
29					
30					

Medication Disposition Record

Date: _____ Quantity Destroyed: _____ Quantity sent with resident: _____

Nurse 1: _____

Nurse 2: _____

Comments: _____

Resident Controlled Substance Record

Resident				Date Received	MD
Medication			Dose	RX#	Nurse receiving
Directions for medication (May place pharmacy Label)				Amount received	2nd Nurse signature

#	Date	Time	Amount Given	Nurse Signature	Amount Remaining
1					
2					
3					
4					
5					
6					
7					
8					
9					
10					
11					
12					
13					
14					
15					
16					
17					
18					
19					
20					
21					
22					
23					
24					
25					
26					
27					
28					
29					
30					

Medication Disposition Record

Date: _____ Quantity Destroyed: _____ Quantity sent with resident: _____

Nurse 1: _____

Nurse 2: _____

Comments: _____

Resident Controlled Substance Record

Resident					Date Received	MD	
Medication				Dose	RX#	Nurse receiving	
Directions for medication (May place pharmacy Label)					Amount received	2nd Nurse signature	

#	Date	Time	Amount Given	Nurse Signature	Amount Remaining
1					
2					
3					
4					
5					
6					
7					
8					
9					
10					
11					
12					
13					
14					
15					
16					
17					
18					
19					
20					
21					
22					
23					
24					
25					
26					
27					
28					
29					
30					

Medication Disposition Record

Date: _____ Quantity Destroyed: _____ Quantity sent with resident: _____

Nurse 1: _____

Nurse 2: _____

Comments: _____

Resident Controlled Substance Record

Resident				Date Received	MD	
Medication			Dose	RX#	Nurse receiving	
Directions for medication (May place pharmacy Label)				Amount received	2nd Nurse signature	

#	Date	Time	Amount Given	Nurse Signature	Amount Remaining
1					
2					
3					
4					
5					
6					
7					
8					
9					
10					
11					
12					
13					
14					
15					
16					
17					
18					
19					
20					
21					
22					
23					
24					
25					
26					
27					
28					
29					
30					

Medication Disposition Record

Date: _____ Quantity Destroyed: _____ Quantity sent with resident: _____

Nurse 1: _____

Nurse 2: _____

Comments: _____

Resident Controlled Substance Record

Resident				Date Received	MD	
Medication			Dose	RX#	Nurse receiving	
Directions for medication (May place pharmacy Label)				Amount received	2nd Nurse signature	

#	Date	Time	Amount Given	Nurse Signature	Amount Remaining
1					
2					
3					
4					
5					
6					
7					
8					
9					
10					
11					
12					
13					
14					
15					
16					
17					
18					
19					
20					
21					
22					
23					
24					
25					
26					
27					
28					
29					
30					

Medication Disposition Record

Date: _____ Quantity Destroyed: _____ Quantity sent with resident: _____

Nurse 1: _____

Nurse 2: _____

Comments: _____

Resident Controlled Substance Record

Resident			Date Received	MD	
Medication		Dose	RX#	Nurse receiving	
Directions for medication (May place pharmacy Label)			Amount received	2nd Nurse signature	

#	Date	Time	Amount Given	Nurse Signature	Amount Remaining
1					
2					
3					
4					
5					
6					
7					
8					
9					
10					
11					
12					
13					
14					
15					
16					
17					
18					
19					
20					
21					
22					
23					
24					
25					
26					
27					
28					
29					
30					

Medication Disposition Record

Date: _____ Quantity Destroyed: _____ Quantity sent with resident: _____

Nurse 1: _____

Nurse 2: _____

Comments: _____

Resident Controlled Substance Record

Resident				Date Received	MD	
Medication			Dose	RX#	Nurse receiving	
Directions for medication (May place pharmacy Label)				Amount received	2nd Nurse signature	

#	Date	Time	Amount Given	Nurse Signature	Amount Remaining
1					
2					
3					
4					
5					
6					
7					
8					
9					
10					
11					
12					
13					
14					
15					
16					
17					
18					
19					
20					
21					
22					
23					
24					
25					
26					
27					
28					
29					
30					

Medication Disposition Record

Date: _____ Quantity Destroyed: _____ Quantity sent with resident: _____

Nurse 1: _____

Nurse 2: _____

Comments: _____

Resident Controlled Substance Record

Resident				Date Received	MD	
Medication			Dose	RX#	Nurse receiving	
Directions for medication (May place pharmacy Label)				Amount received	2nd Nurse signature	

#	Date	Time	Amount Given	Nurse Signature	Amount Remaining
1					
2					
3					
4					
5					
6					
7					
8					
9					
10					
11					
12					
13					
14					
15					
16					
17					
18					
19					
20					
21					
22					
23					
24					
25					
26					
27					
28					
29					
30					

Medication Disposition Record

Date: _____ Quantity Destroyed: _____ Quantity sent with resident: _____

Nurse 1: _____

Nurse 2: _____

Comments: _____

Resident Controlled Substance Record

Resident		Date Received	MD
Medication	Dose	RX#	Nurse receiving
Directions for medication (May place pharmacy Label)		Amount received	2nd Nurse signature

#	Date	Time	Amount Given	Nurse Signature	Amount Remaining
1					
2					
3					
4					
5					
6					
7					
8					
9					
10					
11					
12					
13					
14					
15					
16					
17					
18					
19					
20					
21					
22					
23					
24					
25					
26					
27					
28					
29					
30					

Medication Disposition Record

Date: _____ Quantity Destroyed: _____ Quantity sent with resident: _____

Nurse 1: _____

Nurse 2: _____

Comments: _____

Resident Controlled Substance Record

Resident				Date Received	MD	
Medication			Dose	RX#	Nurse receiving	
Directions for medication (May place pharmacy Label)				Amount received	2nd Nurse signature	

#	Date	Time	Amount Given	Nurse Signature	Amount Remaining
1					
2					
3					
4					
5					
6					
7					
8					
9					
10					
11					
12					
13					
14					
15					
16					
17					
18					
19					
20					
21					
22					
23					
24					
25					
26					
27					
28					
29					
30					

Medication Disposition Record

Date: _____ Quantity Destroyed: _____ Quantity sent with resident: _____

Nurse 1: _____

Nurse 2: _____

Comments: _____

Resident Controlled Substance Record

Resident					Date Received		MD	
Medication				Dose	RX#		Nurse receiving	
Directions for medication (May place pharmacy Label)					Amount received		2nd Nurse signature	

#	Date	Time	Amount Given	Nurse Signature	Amount Remaining
1					
2					
3					
4					
5					
6					
7					
8					
9					
10					
11					
12					
13					
14					
15					
16					
17					
18					
19					
20					
21					
22					
23					
24					
25					
26					
27					
28					
29					
30					

Medication Disposition Record

Date: _____ Quantity Destroyed: _____ Quantity sent with resident: _____

Nurse 1: _____

Nurse 2: _____

Comments: _____

Resident Controlled Substance Record

Resident			Date Received	MD	
Medication		Dose	RX#	Nurse receiving	
Directions for medication (May place pharmacy Label)			Amount received	2nd Nurse signature	

#	Date	Time	Amount Given	Nurse Signature	Amount Remaining
1					
2					
3					
4					
5					
6					
7					
8					
9					
10					
11					
12					
13					
14					
15					
16					
17					
18					
19					
20					
21					
22					
23					
24					
25					
26					
27					
28					
29					
30					

Medication Disposition Record

Date: _____ Quantity Destroyed: _____ Quantity sent with resident: _____

Nurse 1: _____

Nurse 2: _____

Comments: _____

Resident Controlled Substance Record

Resident				Date Received	MD	
Medication			Dose	RX#	Nurse receiving	
Directions for medication (May place pharmacy Label)				Amount received	2nd Nurse signature	

#	Date	Time	Amount Given	Nurse Signature	Amount Remaining
1					
2					
3					
4					
5					
6					
7					
8					
9					
10					
11					
12					
13					
14					
15					
16					
17					
18					
19					
20					
21					
22					
23					
24					
25					
26					
27					
28					
29					
30					

Medication Disposition Record

Date: _____ Quantity Destroyed: _____ Quantity sent with resident: _____

Nurse 1: _____

Nurse 2: _____

Comments: _____

Resident Controlled Substance Record

Resident		Date Received	MD

Medication	Dose	RX#	Nurse receiving

Directions for medication (May place pharmacy Label)	Amount received	2nd Nurse signature

#	Date	Time	Amount Given	Nurse Signature	Amount Remaining
1					
2					
3					
4					
5					
6					
7					
8					
9					
10					
11					
12					
13					
14					
15					
16					
17					
18					
19					
20					
21					
22					
23					
24					
25					
26					
27					
28					
29					
30					

Medication Disposition Record

Date: _____ Quantity Destroyed: _____ Quantity sent with resident: _____

Nurse 1: _____

Nurse 2: _____

Comments: _____

Resident Controlled Substance Record

Resident				Date Received	MD	
Medication			Dose	RX#	Nurse receiving	
Directions for medication (May place pharmacy Label)				Amount received	2nd Nurse signature	

#	Date	Time	Amount Given	Nurse Signature	Amount Remaining
1					
2					
3					
4					
5					
6					
7					
8					
9					
10					
11					
12					
13					
14					
15					
16					
17					
18					
19					
20					
21					
22					
23					
24					
25					
26					
27					
28					
29					
30					

Medication Disposition Record

Date: _____ Quantity Destroyed: _____ Quantity sent with resident: _____

Nurse 1: _____

Nurse 2: _____

Comments: _____

Resident Controlled Substance Record

Resident				Date Received	MD	
Medication			Dose	RX#	Nurse receiving	
Directions for medication (May place pharmacy Label)				Amount received	2nd Nurse signature	

#	Date	Time	Amount Given	Nurse Signature	Amount Remaining
1					
2					
3					
4					
5					
6					
7					
8					
9					
10					
11					
12					
13					
14					
15					
16					
17					
18					
19					
20					
21					
22					
23					
24					
25					
26					
27					
28					
29					
30					

Medication Disposition Record

Date: _____ Quantity Destroyed: _____ Quantity sent with resident: _____

Nurse 1: _____

Nurse 2: _____

Comments: _____

Resident Controlled Substance Record

Resident				Date Received	MD	
Medication			Dose	RX#	Nurse receiving	
Directions for medication (May place pharmacy Label)				Amount received	2nd Nurse signature	

#	Date	Time	Amount Given	Nurse Signature	Amount Remaining
1					
2					
3					
4					
5					
6					
7					
8					
9					
10					
11					
12					
13					
14					
15					
16					
17					
18					
19					
20					
21					
22					
23					
24					
25					
26					
27					
28					
29					
30					

Medication Disposition Record

Date: _____ Quantity Destroyed: _____ Quantity sent with resident: _____

Nurse 1: _____

Nurse 2: _____

Comments: _____

Resident Controlled Substance Record

Resident			Date Received	MD
Medication		Dose	RX#	Nurse receiving
Directions for medication (May place pharmacy Label)			Amount received	2nd Nurse signature

#	Date	Time	Amount Given	Nurse Signature	Amount Remaining
1					
2					
3					
4					
5					
6					
7					
8					
9					
10					
11					
12					
13					
14					
15					
16					
17					
18					
19					
20					
21					
22					
23					
24					
25					
26					
27					
28					
29					
30					

Medication Disposition Record

Date: _____ Quantity Destroyed: _____ Quantity sent with resident: _____

Nurse 1: _____

Nurse 2: _____

Comments: _____

Resident Controlled Substance Record

Resident					Date Received	MD	
Medication				Dose	RX#	Nurse receiving	
Directions for medication (May place pharmacy Label)					Amount received	2nd Nurse signature	

#	Date	Time	Amount Given	Nurse Signature	Amount Remaining
1					
2					
3					
4					
5					
6					
7					
8					
9					
10					
11					
12					
13					
14					
15					
16					
17					
18					
19					
20					
21					
22					
23					
24					
25					
26					
27					
28					
29					
30					

Medication Disposition Record

Date: _____ Quantity Destroyed: _____ Quantity sent with resident: _____

Nurse 1: _____

Nurse 2: _____

Comments: _____

Resident Controlled Substance Record

Resident					Date Received	MD	
Medication				Dose	RX#	Nurse receiving	
Directions for medication (May place pharmacy Label)					Amount received	2nd Nurse signature	

#	Date	Time	Amount Given	Nurse Signature	Amount Remaining
1					
2					
3					
4					
5					
6					
7					
8					
9					
10					
11					
12					
13					
14					
15					
16					
17					
18					
19					
20					
21					
22					
23					
24					
25					
26					
27					
28					
29					
30					

Medication Disposition Record

Date: _____ Quantity Destroyed: _____ Quantity sent with resident: _____

Nurse 1: _____

Nurse 2: _____

Comments: _____

Resident Controlled Substance Record

Resident				Date Received		MD	

Medication			Dose	RX#		Nurse receiving	

Directions for medication (May place pharmacy Label)				Amount received		2nd Nurse signature	

#	Date	Time	Amount Given	Nurse Signature	Amount Remaining
1					
2					
3					
4					
5					
6					
7					
8					
9					
10					
11					
12					
13					
14					
15					
16					
17					
18					
19					
20					
21					
22					
23					
24					
25					
26					
27					
28					
29					
30					

Medication Disposition Record

Date: _____ Quantity Destroyed: _____ Quantity sent with resident: _____

Nurse 1: _____

Nurse 2: _____

Comments: _____

Resident Controlled Substance Record

Resident		Date Received	MD

Medication	Dose	RX#	Nurse receiving

Directions for medication (May place pharmacy Label)	Amount received	2nd Nurse signature

#	Date	Time	Amount Given	Nurse Signature	Amount Remaining
1					
2					
3					
4					
5					
6					
7					
8					
9					
10					
11					
12					
13					
14					
15					
16					
17					
18					
19					
20					
21					
22					
23					
24					
25					
26					
27					
28					
29					
30					

Medication Disposition Record

Date: _____ Quantity Destroyed: _____ Quantity sent with resident: _____

Nurse 1: _____

Nurse 2: _____

Comments: _____

Resident Controlled Substance Record

Resident			Date Received	MD	
Medication		Dose	RX#	Nurse receiving	
Directions for medication (May place pharmacy Label)			Amount received	2nd Nurse signature	

#	Date	Time	Amount Given	Nurse Signature	Amount Remaining
1					
2					
3					
4					
5					
6					
7					
8					
9					
10					
11					
12					
13					
14					
15					
16					
17					
18					
19					
20					
21					
22					
23					
24					
25					
26					
27					
28					
29					
30					

Medication Disposition Record

Date: _____ Quantity Destroyed: _____ Quantity sent with resident: _____

Nurse 1: _____

Nurse 2: _____

Comments: _____

Resident Controlled Substance Record

Resident		Date Received	MD
Medication	Dose	RX#	Nurse receiving
Directions for medication (May place pharmacy Label)		Amount received	2nd Nurse signature

#	Date	Time	Amount Given	Nurse Signature	Amount Remaining
1					
2					
3					
4					
5					
6					
7					
8					
9					
10					
11					
12					
13					
14					
15					
16					
17					
18					
19					
20					
21					
22					
23					
24					
25					
26					
27					
28					
29					
30					

Medication Disposition Record

Date: _____ Quantity Destroyed: _____ Quantity sent with resident: _____

Nurse 1: _____

Nurse 2: _____

Comments: _____

Resident Controlled Substance Record

Resident				Date Received	MD	
Medication			Dose	RX#	Nurse receiving	
Directions for medication (May place pharmacy Label)				Amount received	2nd Nurse signature	

#	Date	Time	Amount Given	Nurse Signature	Amount Remaining
1					
2					
3					
4					
5					
6					
7					
8					
9					
10					
11					
12					
13					
14					
15					
16					
17					
18					
19					
20					
21					
22					
23					
24					
25					
26					
27					
28					
29					
30					

Medication Disposition Record

Date: _____ Quantity Destroyed: _____ Quantity sent with resident: _____

Nurse 1: _____

Nurse 2: _____

Comments: _____

Resident Controlled Substance Record

Resident						Date Received	MD	
Medication				Dose		RX#	Nurse receiving	
Directions for medication (May place pharmacy Label)						Amount received	2nd Nurse signature	

#	Date	Time	Amount Given	Nurse Signature	Amount Remaining
1					
2					
3					
4					
5					
6					
7					
8					
9					
10					
11					
12					
13					
14					
15					
16					
17					
18					
19					
20					
21					
22					
23					
24					
25					
26					
27					
28					
29					
30					

Medication Disposition Record

Date: _____ Quantity Destroyed: _____ Quantity sent with resident: _____

Nurse 1: _____

Nurse 2: _____

Comments: _____

Resident Controlled Substance Record

Resident				Date Received	MD	
Medication			Dose	RX#	Nurse receiving	
Directions for medication (May place pharmacy Label)				Amount received	2nd Nurse signature	

#	Date	Time	Amount Given	Nurse Signature	Amount Remaining
1					
2					
3					
4					
5					
6					
7					
8					
9					
10					
11					
12					
13					
14					
15					
16					
17					
18					
19					
20					
21					
22					
23					
24					
25					
26					
27					
28					
29					
30					

Medication Disposition Record

Date: _____ Quantity Destroyed: _____ Quantity sent with resident: _____

Nurse 1: _____

Nurse 2: _____

Comments: _____

Resident Controlled Substance Record

Resident					Date Received	MD	

Medication			Dose	RX#	Nurse receiving	

Directions for medication (May place pharmacy Label)				Amount received	2nd Nurse signature	

#	Date	Time	Amount Given	Nurse Signature	Amount Remaining
1					
2					
3					
4					
5					
6					
7					
8					
9					
10					
11					
12					
13					
14					
15					
16					
17					
18					
19					
20					
21					
22					
23					
24					
25					
26					
27					
28					
29					
30					

Medication Disposition Record

Date: _____ Quantity Destroyed: _____ Quantity sent with resident: _____

Nurse 1: _____

Nurse 2: _____

Comments: _____

Resident Controlled Substance Record

Resident				Date Received	MD	
Medication			Dose	RX#	Nurse receiving	
Directions for medication (May place pharmacy Label)				Amount received	2nd Nurse signature	

#	Date	Time	Amount Given	Nurse Signature	Amount Remaining
1					
2					
3					
4					
5					
6					
7					
8					
9					
10					
11					
12					
13					
14					
15					
16					
17					
18					
19					
20					
21					
22					
23					
24					
25					
26					
27					
28					
29					
30					

Medication Disposition Record

Date: _____ Quantity Destroyed: _____ Quantity sent with resident: _____

Nurse 1: _____

Nurse 2: _____

Comments: _____

Resident Controlled Substance Record

Resident				Date Received	MD	
Medication			Dose	RX#	Nurse receiving	
Directions for medication (May place pharmacy Label)				Amount received	2nd Nurse signature	

#	Date	Time	Amount Given	Nurse Signature	Amount Remaining
1					
2					
3					
4					
5					
6					
7					
8					
9					
10					
11					
12					
13					
14					
15					
16					
17					
18					
19					
20					
21					
22					
23					
24					
25					
26					
27					
28					
29					
30					

Medication Disposition Record

Date: _____ Quantity Destroyed: _____ Quantity sent with resident: _____

Nurse 1: _____

Nurse 2: _____

Comments: _____

Resident Controlled Substance Record

Resident				Date Received	MD	
Medication			Dose	RX#	Nurse receiving	
Directions for medication (May place pharmacy Label)				Amount received	2nd Nurse signature	

#	Date	Time	Amount Given	Nurse Signature	Amount Remaining
1					
2					
3					
4					
5					
6					
7					
8					
9					
10					
11					
12					
13					
14					
15					
16					
17					
18					
19					
20					
21					
22					
23					
24					
25					
26					
27					
28					
29					
30					

Medication Disposition Record

Date: _____ Quantity Destroyed: _____ Quantity sent with resident: _____

Nurse 1: _____

Nurse 2: _____

Comments: _____

Resident Controlled Substance Record

Resident				Date Received	MD	
Medication			Dose	RX#	Nurse receiving	
Directions for medication (May place pharmacy Label)				Amount received	2nd Nurse signature	

#	Date	Time	Amount Given	Nurse Signature	Amount Remaining
1					
2					
3					
4					
5					
6					
7					
8					
9					
10					
11					
12					
13					
14					
15					
16					
17					
18					
19					
20					
21					
22					
23					
24					
25					
26					
27					
28					
29					
30					

Medication Disposition Record

Date: _____ Quantity Destroyed: _____ Quantity sent with resident: _____

Nurse 1: _____

Nurse 2: _____

Comments: _____

Resident Controlled Substance Record

Resident				Date Received	MD	
Medication			Dose	RX#	Nurse receiving	
Directions for medication (May place pharmacy Label)				Amount received	2nd Nurse signature	

#	Date	Time	Amount Given	Nurse Signature	Amount Remaining
1					
2					
3					
4					
5					
6					
7					
8					
9					
10					
11					
12					
13					
14					
15					
16					
17					
18					
19					
20					
21					
22					
23					
24					
25					
26					
27					
28					
29					
30					

Medication Disposition Record

Date: _____ Quantity Destroyed: _____ Quantity sent with resident: _____

Nurse 1: _____

Nurse 2: _____

Comments: _____

Resident Controlled Substance Record

Resident				Date Received	MD
Medication			Dose	RX#	Nurse receiving
Directions for medication (May place pharmacy Label)				Amount received	2nd Nurse signature

#	Date	Time	Amount Given	Nurse Signature	Amount Remaining
1					
2					
3					
4					
5					
6					
7					
8					
9					
10					
11					
12					
13					
14					
15					
16					
17					
18					
19					
20					
21					
22					
23					
24					
25					
26					
27					
28					
29					
30					

Medication Disposition Record

Date: _____ Quantity Destroyed: _____ Quantity sent with resident: _____

Nurse 1: _____

Nurse 2: _____

Comments: _____

Resident Controlled Substance Record

Resident					Date Received	MD	
Medication				Dose	RX#	Nurse receiving	
Directions for medication (May place pharmacy Label)					Amount received	2nd Nurse signature	

#	Date	Time	Amount Given	Nurse Signature	Amount Remaining
1					
2					
3					
4					
5					
6					
7					
8					
9					
10					
11					
12					
13					
14					
15					
16					
17					
18					
19					
20					
21					
22					
23					
24					
25					
26					
27					
28					
29					
30					

Medication Disposition Record

Date: _____ Quantity Destroyed: _____ Quantity sent with resident: _____

Nurse 1: _____

Nurse 2: _____

Comments: _____

Resident Controlled Substance Record

Resident				Date Received	MD	
Medication			Dose	RX#	Nurse receiving	
Directions for medication (May place pharmacy Label)				Amount received	2nd Nurse signature	

#	Date	Time	Amount Given	Nurse Signature	Amount Remaining
1					
2					
3					
4					
5					
6					
7					
8					
9					
10					
11					
12					
13					
14					
15					
16					
17					
18					
19					
20					
21					
22					
23					
24					
25					
26					
27					
28					
29					
30					

Medication Disposition Record

Date: _____ Quantity Destroyed: _____ Quantity sent with resident: _____

Nurse 1: _____

Nurse 2: _____

Comments: _____

Resident Controlled Substance Record

Resident				Date Received	MD
Medication			Dose	RX#	Nurse receiving
Directions for medication (May place pharmacy Label)				Amount received	2nd Nurse signature

#	Date	Time	Amount Given	Nurse Signature	Amount Remaining
1					
2					
3					
4					
5					
6					
7					
8					
9					
10					
11					
12					
13					
14					
15					
16					
17					
18					
19					
20					
21					
22					
23					
24					
25					
26					
27					
28					
29					
30					

Medication Disposition Record

Date: _____ Quantity Destroyed: _____ Quantity sent with resident: _____

Nurse 1: _____

Nurse 2: _____

Comments: _____

Resident Controlled Substance Record

Resident				Date Received	MD
Medication			Dose	RX#	Nurse receiving
Directions for medication (May place pharmacy Label)				Amount received	2nd Nurse signature

#	Date	Time	Amount Given	Nurse Signature	Amount Remaining
1					
2					
3					
4					
5					
6					
7					
8					
9					
10					
11					
12					
13					
14					
15					
16					
17					
18					
19					
20					
21					
22					
23					
24					
25					
26					
27					
28					
29					
30					

Medication Disposition Record

Date: _____ Quantity Destroyed: _____ Quantity sent with resident: _____

Nurse 1: _____

Nurse 2: _____

Comments: _____

Resident Controlled Substance Record

Resident			Date Received	MD	
Medication		Dose	RX#	Nurse receiving	
Directions for medication (May place pharmacy Label)			Amount received	2nd Nurse signature	

#	Date	Time	Amount Given	Nurse Signature	Amount Remaining
1					
2					
3					
4					
5					
6					
7					
8					
9					
10					
11					
12					
13					
14					
15					
16					
17					
18					
19					
20					
21					
22					
23					
24					
25					
26					
27					
28					
29					
30					

Medication Disposition Record

Date: _____ Quantity Destroyed: _____ Quantity sent with resident: _____

Nurse 1: _____

Nurse 2: _____

Comments: _____

Resident Controlled Substance Record

Resident			Date Received	MD	
Medication		Dose	RX#	Nurse receiving	
Directions for medication (May place pharmacy Label)			Amount received	2nd Nurse signature	

#	Date	Time	Amount Given	Nurse Signature	Amount Remaining
1					
2					
3					
4					
5					
6					
7					
8					
9					
10					
11					
12					
13					
14					
15					
16					
17					
18					
19					
20					
21					
22					
23					
24					
25					
26					
27					
28					
29					
30					

Medication Disposition Record

Date: _____ Quantity Destroyed: _____ Quantity sent with resident: _____

Nurse 1: _____

Nurse 2: _____

Comments: _____

Resident Controlled Substance Record

Resident				Date Received	MD	
Medication			Dose	RX#	Nurse receiving	
Directions for medication (May place pharmacy Label)				Amount received	2nd Nurse signature	

#	Date	Time	Amount Given	Nurse Signature	Amount Remaining
1					
2					
3					
4					
5					
6					
7					
8					
9					
10					
11					
12					
13					
14					
15					
16					
17					
18					
19					
20					
21					
22					
23					
24					
25					
26					
27					
28					
29					
30					

Medication Disposition Record

Date: _____ Quantity Destroyed: _____ Quantity sent with resident: _____

Nurse 1: _____

Nurse 2: _____

Comments: _____

Resident Controlled Substance Record

Resident					Date Received	MD	
Medication				Dose	RX#	Nurse receiving	
Directions for medication (May place pharmacy Label)					Amount received	2nd Nurse signature	

#	Date	Time	Amount Given	Nurse Signature	Amount Remaining
1					
2					
3					
4					
5					
6					
7					
8					
9					
10					
11					
12					
13					
14					
15					
16					
17					
18					
19					
20					
21					
22					
23					
24					
25					
26					
27					
28					
29					
30					

Medication Disposition Record

Date: _____ Quantity Destroyed: _____ Quantity sent with resident: _____

Nurse 1: _____

Nurse 2: _____

Comments: _____

Resident Controlled Substance Record

Resident			Date Received	MD	
Medication		Dose	RX#	Nurse receiving	
Directions for medication (May place pharmacy Label)			Amount received	2nd Nurse signature	

#	Date	Time	Amount Given	Nurse Signature	Amount Remaining
1					
2					
3					
4					
5					
6					
7					
8					
9					
10					
11					
12					
13					
14					
15					
16					
17					
18					
19					
20					
21					
22					
23					
24					
25					
26					
27					
28					
29					
30					

Medication Disposition Record

Date: _____ Quantity Destroyed: _____ Quantity sent with resident: _____

Nurse 1: _____

Nurse 2: _____

Comments: _____

Resident Controlled Substance Record

Resident			Date Received	MD	
Medication		Dose	RX#	Nurse receiving	
Directions for medication (May place pharmacy Label)			Amount received	2nd Nurse signature	

#	Date	Time	Amount Given	Nurse Signature	Amount Remaining
1					
2					
3					
4					
5					
6					
7					
8					
9					
10					
11					
12					
13					
14					
15					
16					
17					
18					
19					
20					
21					
22					
23					
24					
25					
26					
27					
28					
29					
30					

Medication Disposition Record

Date: _____ Quantity Destroyed: _____ Quantity sent with resident: _____

Nurse 1: _____

Nurse 2: _____

Comments: _____

Resident Controlled Substance Record

Resident					Date Received	MD	
Medication				Dose	RX#	Nurse receiving	
Directions for medication (May place pharmacy Label)					Amount received	2nd Nurse signature	

#	Date	Time	Amount Given	Nurse Signature	Amount Remaining
1					
2					
3					
4					
5					
6					
7					
8					
9					
10					
11					
12					
13					
14					
15					
16					
17					
18					
19					
20					
21					
22					
23					
24					
25					
26					
27					
28					
29					
30					

Medication Disposition Record

Date: _____ Quantity Destroyed: _____ Quantity sent with resident: _____

Nurse 1: _____

Nurse 2: _____

Comments: _____

Resident Controlled Substance Record

Resident				Date Received	MD	
Medication			Dose	RX#	Nurse receiving	
Directions for medication (May place pharmacy Label)				Amount received	2nd Nurse signature	

#	Date	Time	Amount Given	Nurse Signature	Amount Remaining
1					
2					
3					
4					
5					
6					
7					
8					
9					
10					
11					
12					
13					
14					
15					
16					
17					
18					
19					
20					
21					
22					
23					
24					
25					
26					
27					
28					
29					
30					

Medication Disposition Record

Date: _____ Quantity Destroyed: _____ Quantity sent with resident: _____

Nurse 1: _____

Nurse 2: _____

Comments: _____

Resident Controlled Substance Record

Resident					Date Received	MD	
Medication				Dose	RX#	Nurse receiving	
Directions for medication (May place pharmacy Label)					Amount received	2nd Nurse signature	

#	Date	Time	Amount Given	Nurse Signature	Amount Remaining
1					
2					
3					
4					
5					
6					
7					
8					
9					
10					
11					
12					
13					
14					
15					
16					
17					
18					
19					
20					
21					
22					
23					
24					
25					
26					
27					
28					
29					
30					

Medication Disposition Record

Date: _____ Quantity Destroyed: _____ Quantity sent with resident: _____

Nurse 1: _____

Nurse 2: _____

Comments: _____

Resident Controlled Substance Record

Resident				Date Received	MD	
Medication			Dose	RX#	Nurse receiving	
Directions for medication (May place pharmacy Label)				Amount received	2nd Nurse signature	

#	Date	Time	Amount Given	Nurse Signature	Amount Remaining
1					
2					
3					
4					
5					
6					
7					
8					
9					
10					
11					
12					
13					
14					
15					
16					
17					
18					
19					
20					
21					
22					
23					
24					
25					
26					
27					
28					
29					
30					

Medication Disposition Record

Date: _____ Quantity Destroyed: _____ Quantity sent with resident: _____

Nurse 1: _____

Nurse 2: _____

Comments: _____

Resident Controlled Substance Record

Resident				Date Received	MD
Medication			Dose	RX#	Nurse receiving
Directions for medication (May place pharmacy Label)				Amount received	2nd Nurse signature

#	Date	Time	Amount Given	Nurse Signature	Amount Remaining
1					
2					
3					
4					
5					
6					
7					
8					
9					
10					
11					
12					
13					
14					
15					
16					
17					
18					
19					
20					
21					
22					
23					
24					
25					
26					
27					
28					
29					
30					

Medication Disposition Record

Date: _____ Quantity Destroyed: _____ Quantity sent with resident: _____

Nurse 1: _____

Nurse 2: _____

Comments: _____

Resident Controlled Substance Record

Resident		Date Received	MD

Medication	Dose	RX#	Nurse receiving

Directions for medication (May place pharmacy Label)	Amount received	2nd Nurse signature

#	Date	Time	Amount Given	Nurse Signature	Amount Remaining
1					
2					
3					
4					
5					
6					
7					
8					
9					
10					
11					
12					
13					
14					
15					
16					
17					
18					
19					
20					
21					
22					
23					
24					
25					
26					
27					
28					
29					
30					

Medication Disposition Record

Date: _____ Quantity Destroyed: _____ Quantity sent with resident: _____

Nurse 1: _____

Nurse 2: _____

Comments: _____

Resident Controlled Substance Record

Resident					Date Received	MD	
Medication				Dose	RX#	Nurse receiving	
Directions for medication (May place pharmacy Label)					Amount received	2nd Nurse signature	

#	Date	Time	Amount Given	Nurse Signature	Amount Remaining
1					
2					
3					
4					
5					
6					
7					
8					
9					
10					
11					
12					
13					
14					
15					
16					
17					
18					
19					
20					
21					
22					
23					
24					
25					
26					
27					
28					
29					
30					

Medication Disposition Record

Date: _____ Quantity Destroyed: _____ Quantity sent with resident: _____

Nurse 1: _____

Nurse 2: _____

Comments: _____

Resident Controlled Substance Record

Resident			Date Received	MD	
Medication		Dose	RX#	Nurse receiving	
Directions for medication (May place pharmacy Label)			Amount received	2nd Nurse signature	

#	Date	Time	Amount Given	Nurse Signature	Amount Remaining
1					
2					
3					
4					
5					
6					
7					
8					
9					
10					
11					
12					
13					
14					
15					
16					
17					
18					
19					
20					
21					
22					
23					
24					
25					
26					
27					
28					
29					
30					

Medication Disposition Record

Date: _____ Quantity Destroyed: _____ Quantity sent with resident: _____

Nurse 1: _____

Nurse 2: _____

Comments: _____

Resident Controlled Substance Record

Resident				Date Received	MD	

Medication			Dose	RX#	Nurse receiving	

Directions for medication (May place pharmacy Label)				Amount received	2nd Nurse signature	

#	Date	Time	Amount Given	Nurse Signature	Amount Remaining
1					
2					
3					
4					
5					
6					
7					
8					
9					
10					
11					
12					
13					
14					
15					
16					
17					
18					
19					
20					
21					
22					
23					
24					
25					
26					
27					
28					
29					
30					

Medication Disposition Record

Date: _____ Quantity Destroyed: _____ Quantity sent with resident: _____

Nurse 1: _____

Nurse 2: _____

Comments: _____

Resident Controlled Substance Record

Resident		Date Received	MD

Medication	Dose	RX#	Nurse receiving

Directions for medication (May place pharmacy Label)	Amount received	2nd Nurse signature

#	Date	Time	Amount Given	Nurse Signature	Amount Remaining
1					
2					
3					
4					
5					
6					
7					
8					
9					
10					
11					
12					
13					
14					
15					
16					
17					
18					
19					
20					
21					
22					
23					
24					
25					
26					
27					
28					
29					
30					

Medication Disposition Record

Date: _____ Quantity Destroyed: _____ Quantity sent with resident: _____

Nurse 1: _____

Nurse 2: _____

Comments: _____

Resident Controlled Substance Record

Resident			Date Received	MD
Medication		Dose	RX#	Nurse receiving
Directions for medication (May place pharmacy Label)			Amount received	2nd Nurse signature

#	Date	Time	Amount Given	Nurse Signature	Amount Remaining
1					
2					
3					
4					
5					
6					
7					
8					
9					
10					
11					
12					
13					
14					
15					
16					
17					
18					
19					
20					
21					
22					
23					
24					
25					
26					
27					
28					
29					
30					

Medication Disposition Record

Date: _____ Quantity Destroyed: _____ Quantity sent with resident: _____

Nurse 1: _____

Nurse 2: _____

Comments: _____

Resident Controlled Substance Record

Resident			Date Received	MD	
Medication		Dose	RX#	Nurse receiving	
Directions for medication (May place pharmacy Label)			Amount received	2nd Nurse signature	

#	Date	Time	Amount Given	Nurse Signature	Amount Remaining
1					
2					
3					
4					
5					
6					
7					
8					
9					
10					
11					
12					
13					
14					
15					
16					
17					
18					
19					
20					
21					
22					
23					
24					
25					
26					
27					
28					
29					
30					

Medication Disposition Record

Date: _____ Quantity Destroyed: _____ Quantity sent with resident: _____

Nurse 1: _____

Nurse 2: _____

Comments: _____

Resident Controlled Substance Record

Resident			Date Received	MD	
Medication		Dose	RX#	Nurse receiving	
Directions for medication (May place pharmacy Label)			Amount received	2nd Nurse signature	

#	Date	Time	Amount Given	Nurse Signature	Amount Remaining
1					
2					
3					
4					
5					
6					
7					
8					
9					
10					
11					
12					
13					
14					
15					
16					
17					
18					
19					
20					
21					
22					
23					
24					
25					
26					
27					
28					
29					
30					

Medication Disposition Record

Date: _____ Quantity Destroyed: _____ Quantity sent with resident: _____

Nurse 1: _____

Nurse 2: _____

Comments: _____

Resident Controlled Substance Record

Resident			Date Received	MD
Medication		Dose	RX#	Nurse receiving
Directions for medication (May place pharmacy Label)			Amount received	2nd Nurse signature

#	Date	Time	Amount Given	Nurse Signature	Amount Remaining
1					
2					
3					
4					
5					
6					
7					
8					
9					
10					
11					
12					
13					
14					
15					
16					
17					
18					
19					
20					
21					
22					
23					
24					
25					
26					
27					
28					
29					
30					

Medication Disposition Record

Date: _____ Quantity Destroyed: _____ Quantity sent with resident: _____

Nurse 1: _____

Nurse 2: _____

Comments: _____

Resident Controlled Substance Record

Resident			Date Received	MD
Medication		Dose	RX#	Nurse receiving
Directions for medication (May place pharmacy Label)			Amount received	2nd Nurse signature

#	Date	Time	Amount Given	Nurse Signature	Amount Remaining
1					
2					
3					
4					
5					
6					
7					
8					
9					
10					
11					
12					
13					
14					
15					
16					
17					
18					
19					
20					
21					
22					
23					
24					
25					
26					
27					
28					
29					
30					

Medication Disposition Record

Date: _____ Quantity Destroyed: _____ Quantity sent with resident: _____

Nurse 1: _____

Nurse 2: _____

Comments: _____

Resident Controlled Substance Record

Resident		Date Received	MD

Medication	Dose	RX#	Nurse receiving

Directions for medication (May place pharmacy Label)	Amount received	2nd Nurse signature

#	Date	Time	Amount Given	Nurse Signature	Amount Remaining
1					
2					
3					
4					
5					
6					
7					
8					
9					
10					
11					
12					
13					
14					
15					
16					
17					
18					
19					
20					
21					
22					
23					
24					
25					
26					
27					
28					
29					
30					

Medication Disposition Record

Date: _____ Quantity Destroyed: _____ Quantity sent with resident: _____

Nurse 1: _____

Nurse 2: _____

Comments: _____

Resident Controlled Substance Record

Resident				Date Received	MD	
Medication			Dose	RX#	Nurse receiving	
Directions for medication (May place pharmacy Label)				Amount received	2nd Nurse signature	

#	Date	Time	Amount Given	Nurse Signature	Amount Remaining
1					
2					
3					
4					
5					
6					
7					
8					
9					
10					
11					
12					
13					
14					
15					
16					
17					
18					
19					
20					
21					
22					
23					
24					
25					
26					
27					
28					
29					
30					

Medication Disposition Record

Date: _____ Quantity Destroyed: _____ Quantity sent with resident: _____

Nurse 1: _____

Nurse 2: _____

Comments: _____

Resident Controlled Substance Record

Resident				Date Received	MD	
Medication			Dose	RX#	Nurse receiving	
Directions for medication (May place pharmacy Label)				Amount received	2nd Nurse signature	

#	Date	Time	Amount Given	Nurse Signature	Amount Remaining
1					
2					
3					
4					
5					
6					
7					
8					
9					
10					
11					
12					
13					
14					
15					
16					
17					
18					
19					
20					
21					
22					
23					
24					
25					
26					
27					
28					
29					
30					

Medication Disposition Record

Date: _____ Quantity Destroyed: _____ Quantity sent with resident: _____

Nurse 1: _____

Nurse 2: _____

Comments: _____

Resident Controlled Substance Record

Resident			Date Received	MD	
Medication		Dose	RX#	Nurse receiving	
Directions for medication (May place pharmacy Label)			Amount received	2nd Nurse signature	

#	Date	Time	Amount Given	Nurse Signature	Amount Remaining
1					
2					
3					
4					
5					
6					
7					
8					
9					
10					
11					
12					
13					
14					
15					
16					
17					
18					
19					
20					
21					
22					
23					
24					
25					
26					
27					
28					
29					
30					

Medication Disposition Record

Date: _____ Quantity Destroyed: _____ Quantity sent with resident: _____

Nurse 1: _____

Nurse 2: _____

Comments: _____

Resident Controlled Substance Record

Resident				Date Received	MD	
Medication			Dose	RX#	Nurse receiving	
Directions for medication (May place pharmacy Label)				Amount received	2nd Nurse signature	

#	Date	Time	Amount Given	Nurse Signature	Amount Remaining
1					
2					
3					
4					
5					
6					
7					
8					
9					
10					
11					
12					
13					
14					
15					
16					
17					
18					
19					
20					
21					
22					
23					
24					
25					
26					
27					
28					
29					
30					

Medication Disposition Record

Date: _____ Quantity Destroyed: _____ Quantity sent with resident: _____

Nurse 1: _____

Nurse 2: _____

Comments: _____

Resident Controlled Substance Record

Resident					Date Received	MD	
Medication				Dose	RX#	Nurse receiving	
Directions for medication (May place pharmacy Label)					Amount received	2nd Nurse signature	

#	Date	Time	Amount Given	Nurse Signature	Amount Remaining
1					
2					
3					
4					
5					
6					
7					
8					
9					
10					
11					
12					
13					
14					
15					
16					
17					
18					
19					
20					
21					
22					
23					
24					
25					
26					
27					
28					
29					
30					

Medication Disposition Record

Date: _____ Quantity Destroyed: _____ Quantity sent with resident: _____

Nurse 1: _____

Nurse 2: _____

Comments: _____

Resident Controlled Substance Record

Resident				Date Received	MD	
Medication			Dose	RX#	Nurse receiving	
Directions for medication (May place pharmacy Label)				Amount received	2nd Nurse signature	

#	Date	Time	Amount Given	Nurse Signature	Amount Remaining
1					
2					
3					
4					
5					
6					
7					
8					
9					
10					
11					
12					
13					
14					
15					
16					
17					
18					
19					
20					
21					
22					
23					
24					
25					
26					
27					
28					
29					
30					

Medication Disposition Record

Date: _____ Quantity Destroyed: _____ Quantity sent with resident: _____

Nurse 1: _____

Nurse 2: _____

Comments: _____

Resident Controlled Substance Record

Resident				Date Received	MD	
Medication			Dose	RX#	Nurse receiving	
Directions for medication (May place pharmacy Label)				Amount received	2nd Nurse signature	

#	Date	Time	Amount Given	Nurse Signature	Amount Remaining
1					
2					
3					
4					
5					
6					
7					
8					
9					
10					
11					
12					
13					
14					
15					
16					
17					
18					
19					
20					
21					
22					
23					
24					
25					
26					
27					
28					
29					
30					

Medication Disposition Record

Date: _____ Quantity Destroyed: _____ Quantity sent with resident: _____

Nurse 1: _____

Nurse 2: _____

Comments: _____

Resident Controlled Substance Record

Resident				Date Received	MD		
Medication			Dose	RX#	Nurse receiving		
Directions for medication (May place pharmacy Label)				Amount received	2nd Nurse signature		

#	Date	Time	Amount Given	Nurse Signature	Amount Remaining
1					
2					
3					
4					
5					
6					
7					
8					
9					
10					
11					
12					
13					
14					
15					
16					
17					
18					
19					
20					
21					
22					
23					
24					
25					
26					
27					
28					
29					
30					

Medication Disposition Record

Date: _____ Quantity Destroyed: _____ Quantity sent with resident: _____

Nurse 1: _____

Nurse 2: _____

Comments: _____

Shift
to
Shift
Count

Nurse to Nurse Controlled Substance Count Verification

Date	Time	Off Going Nurse	On Coming Nurse
Date	Time	Off Going Nurse	On Coming Nurse

Date	Time	Off Going Nurse	On Coming Nurse
Date	Time	Off Going Nurse	On Coming Nurse

Date	Time	Off Going Nurse	On Coming Nurse
Date	Time	Off Going Nurse	On Coming Nurse

Date	Time	Off Going Nurse	On Coming Nurse
Date	Time	Off Going Nurse	On Coming Nurse

Date	Time	Off Going Nurse	On Coming Nurse
Date	Time	Off Going Nurse	On Coming Nurse

Date	Time	Off Going Nurse	On Coming Nurse
Date	Time	Off Going Nurse	On Coming Nurse

Date	Time	Off Going Nurse	On Coming Nurse
Date	Time	Off Going Nurse	On Coming Nurse

Date	Time	Off Going Nurse	On Coming Nurse
Date	Time	Off Going Nurse	On Coming Nurse

Date	Time	Off Going Nurse	On Coming Nurse
Date	Time	Off Going Nurse	On Coming Nurse

www.ingramcontent.com/pod-product-compliance
Lightning Source LLC
Chambersburg PA
CBHW080913170526
45158CB00008B/2091